Ketamine Infusions:
A Patient's Guide

Everything you need to know before
going for Ketamine infusions

By
Berkley Jones

A Patient's Guide To Ketamine Infusions

Disclaimer:

This book **is not meant** to replace the advice of your personal physician or Ketamine Provider. Always discuss everything with your own provider. Never change your medications or treatments without speaking with your own provider.

This book is meant to be used simply as a guide to help you along your journey with suggestions compiled from other patients going through their own Ketamine journey's.

DEDICATION

This book is dedicated to all the amazing Physicians, CRNAs, and Nurse Practitioners who have committed their lives to helping patients. I especially need to thank Dr. Linda Hodges, my friend and mentor, who helped make this book a reality by sharing her knowledge and wisdom with me. Linda, you are an incredible friend and physician and your patients are so lucky to have you!

I also want to thank Dr. Megan Oxley and the rest of the board at The American Society for Ketamine Physicians for all their hard work on behalf of Ketamine patients and providers. I want to say a special thank you to an amazing CRNA KC Brachvogel at The New England Ketamine Clinic for taking extra special care of veterans.

There are so many others I would like to mention here but the list would go on and on so I am just going to end with thanking two very special CRNAs, Tamara Lynn Vaught of the Ketamine Clinic of West Texas and Ivana Mitic of the Baltimore Ketamine Clinic thank you for your friendship, advice and for all you do to help others!!!!

INTRODUCTION

So you've decided to try Ketamine infusions? Congratulations on taking that first big step towards a better tomorrow.

First, a bit of background on Ketamine, it is an old drug that has been in use in human as well as veterinary medicine since the 1960's. It is considered to be very safe and has very few side effects.

Ketamine was originally developed as a safer anesthetic and has been FDA approved as an anesthetic that provides a high level of analgesia (relief from pain) since 1970. It is used in the military and in hospitals around the world.

Unfortunately Ketamine has also been used illegally which has given it somewhat of a reputation as a club drug (which every article you read loves to mention). Truthfully, that should be the last thing mentioned as Ketamine has done incredible things for people in helping to relieve pain and depression symptoms.

This is a starting guide to help you with all you need to know to get started with your infusions.

The information in this book is for those that are new to Ketamine infusions or those that have already gotten infusions but may not know this information, forgot it, or just need a review. I urge you to re-read this book if you think of a new question as the answer might be here.

CHAPTER 1

A General Overview of Ketamine Infusions

~~~~~~~

Ketamine is not a cure for any illness or disease. That is the first, and most important thing you need to know. Ketamine will not cure depression. It will not cure anxiety, PTSD or any other mental health disorder. It also won't cure Complex Regional Pain Syndrome, Fibromyalgia, Neuropathy, Chronic Pain from Lyme disease or any other type of illnesses.

If it is not a cure then what is Ketamine and why should I get infusions?

Ketamine is a tool. It is a medication that can help immensely with pain and depression and other things. Like any other medicine it needs to be used correctly and it needs to keep being given to continue to work. In other words just like your pills or other medications, you have to keep receiving infusions for it to work.

How many infusions does it usually take to work? This depends on why you may be receiving ketamine infusions. One Ketamine infusion to start with by itself will not do very much for any chronic issue. The first infusions need to be done as a set. For mental health six is usually recommended as the minimum amount and they are usually done every other day, or fit into a specific, short time frame - such as within 2-3 weeks Chronic pain infusions are usually done as a set of 5 to 10. Most doctors do them on consecutive days as that seems to be the most effective initial protocol. We will discuss the two different protocols, for mental health and for chronic pain, in greater detail in the next chapter.

What should I expect to feel immediately after my Ketamine Infusions? You won't feel better overnight and might initially feel worse (some providers call this a post infusion flare up).

With low dose infusions for mental health you may feel dizzy and possibly nauseated for a few hours post infusion. Do not plan to drive for at least 12 to 24 hours after your infusion.

If receiving high-dose infusions for pain, expect to feel dizzy and "out of it" or spacey the first few days to a week after infusions. Get plenty of rest and hydration to help you recover. Post infusions flare ups of both pain and or mental health issues are completely normal. It is not unusual to feel less pain and less depression the day you get Ketamine and then crash the next day. Ketamine needs time to reset the receptors in the brain. That does not happen instantly. Everyone is different but for many people it takes about 1 to 2 weeks after infusions start. Some people even take as long as 3 weeks for it to really start kicking in.

Can I stop my pain or depression medication after infusions?

Do not stop taking other medications without discussing this with your doctor first. Suddenly stopping certain medications can have dangerous side effects and you may be required to do a weaning protocol with your doctors help.

There are a lot of questions about which medications have the potential to interfere with Ketamine infusions.

Benzodiazepines (especially the long acting ones like Klonipin (Clonazepam) and Valium (Diazepam)) are thought to interfere with how well ketamine can work for you. . Discuss weaning off these medications prior to starting infusions to get the best possible results from your infusions.

Versed (Midazolam) and Ativan (Lorazepam) are both shorter acting benzodiazepines and seem to cause a little bit less interference if someone absolutely needs something to help them relax through their infusion. We will discuss this more later on. (However if someone is on daily Ativan or any benzodiazepine a weaning protocol, with your doctor's help should be done before starting infusions for best relief.) The jury is still out on how much interference Xanax (Alprazolam) seems to cause vs Ativan (Lorazepam). Again discuss weaning off it with your doctor before starting infusions if you are taking it daily..

Lamictal is thought to to interfere with Ketamine based on anecdotal evidence and individual clinician experience. Latuda has also been seen to possibly interfere with Ketamine. Discuss this possibility with your doctor if you are on any of these meds and discuss weaning down off of them or using the lowest dose possible.

Your physician may also recommend a higher dose of ketamine or more frequent infusions may help overcome some of the effects these drugs can have on the efficacy of the Ketamine infusions.

For mental health, Ketamine will work best when combined with therapy and possibly an antidepressant, but the combination of ketamine with other medications should always be discussed with your physician. Some people can lower the dose of antidepressants they are taking after infusions but again this needs to be done with the approval of your doctor. Ketamine won't heal underlying traumas or other issues you might be fighting. It is a tool to help you in your fight.

CHAPTER 2

What Questions Should I ask My Provider Before Infusions?

~~~~~~~~~

Using Ketamine for mental health and chronic pain is very new. The guidelines have yet to be set in stone. Providers are developing their protocols through seeing what has worked best for their own patients. That means protocols may vary somewhat depending on the treatment center you attend. The guidelines that are compiled in this book are general guidelines used by many of the providers we have met and spoken with. The following are general questions to ask before your treatments.

1. What dosing protocol does the clinic use?

For example, some clinics use a standard dose for everyone based on weight and do not titrate up or down from this dose. Do they have a maximum dose or do they determine it on an individual basis? Ketamine is not a one size fits all like penicillin for example. The dose of Ketamine is calculated according to your weight and the amount of milligrams of Ketamine. Will the clinic be willing to titrate you dose based on YOUR response and side effects? This will be an important question to ask. Again, this will be different based on why you are receiving ketamine, but all clinics should be able to give you an answer to that question.

2. What is the infusion time??

Usually most depression infusions are given over 40-60 minutes and pain infusions are done over 4 hours.

3. What does your doctor do to prevent rising blood pressure during infusions?

Ketamine is known to actually increase blood pressure. Usually, this is a benign elevation, but some patients do require medication to treat this during their infusions. If you are receiving more than 100 mg of Ketamine you should discuss with your doctor being given a drug called Clonidine which prevents changes in your blood pressure during the infusions. If your doctor is one of the few who gives you propofol with your infusions you may not need clonidine, propofol lowers blood pressure as well. There are some doctors who use propofol in their protocol. Please double-check this with your doctor.

4. What does the doctor use if you get agitated during the infusions?

Drugs such as Versed or Ativan are generally reserved for use with the higher ketamine doses given for pain. Since there is some question of benzodiazepines interfering with Ketamine for mental health most of the doctors administering the lower doses for those diagnoses try to avoid giving these drugs. If however, you are getting agitated during the infusions, discuss with your doctor ways to manage it such as trying to slow down the infusion or giving something such as Benadryl which may help you sleep through the infusion. If you absolutely need a benzodiazepine ask your doctor to start with the lowest possible dose and use one of the shorter acting ones.

5. How do they treat or try to prevent nausea from the Ketamine?

Many people get nauseated from ketamine. To reduce nausea: Avoid eating after midnight if you are going for high dose infusions or generally 4 hours before a lower-dose infusion used for mental health. . (Of note - we have had reports of people feeling like their infusions were less effective when they got zofran during their infusions for depression; if you want, you can ask your doctor about alternatives to zofran (only two people out of the several thousand we have spoken with had this occur so it might be a very rare side effect). Zofran does not seem to interfere with the effects for pain.

6. What other medications may be given with Ketamine?

There is proof that adding IV Magnesium will give better pain/depression relief and lengthen the time the Ketamine works. Speak with your doctor about this. Most people get about 2 grams of magnesium per infusion. Magnesium can cause an upset stomach in some people. If it upsets your stomach ask your doctor to try a lower amount in the infusion. There are a few doctors also add Lidocaine to their pain infusions and some patients have reported it helped increase their pain relief. Other patients reported no increased relief but increased post infusion dizziness beyond what they were accustomed to.

7. Even if your doctor doesn't require it every person should:

A. Have a physical exam with lab work prior to their infusions.

B. Many doctors recommend certain blood tests prior to starting infusions. These tests include liver function tests to make sure your liver is healthy since Ketamine is metabolized in the liver. Some doctors may also want a baseline CBC. (Complete Blood Count)

C. It is also recommended to have your thyroid levels checked if you are being treated for depression as thyroid issues can be an underlying cause of depression. Other labs that should be checked for any patient with depression should be Vitamin D level, Vitamin B12 level, and testing for anemia. These tests are especially important for any patients that are vegan or vegetarian, so be sure to tell your doctor about your general diet if you are being treated for mental health issues.

D. Many doctors recommend a baseline EKG be done prior to infusions, especially for the high dose ones.

8. All patients, prior to infusions, should be given a psychiatric clearance by their regular psychiatrist :

A. If someone has Schizophrenia or Schizoaffective disorder Ketamine is normally contraindicated and they should only be given Ketamine with extreme caution under the guidance of a psychiatric expert who knows the patient well.

B. Some doctors also feel it should be used with caution in people who have Bipolar type 1 disorder as there is a potential to cause, or exacerbate, mania. Bipolar patients should get their infusion when they are in a depressive state. There have been some rare Bipolar patients being thrown into a manic state with ketamine infusions. Please stay in close contact with your doctor before and after infusions and make them immediately aware of any unusual side effects you might be having.

For those with Bipolar disorder I am going to mention again that if you are on Lamictal or Latuda or Abilify some research studies have shown these drugs can decrease how well ketamine can work for you. . This is something important to discuss with your doctor. You might either need a higher dose of ketamine or more frequent infusions. You may need to discuss coming off of it totally and trying another mood stabilizer such as lithium. Do Not Stop Taking Any Medications Without Speaking To Your Doctor First!!!

C. Ketamine is not known to help or to worsen ADD/ADHD and it seems to be safe to use in people with ADD/ADHD and depression. However it does seem from clinician and patient reports that people with ADD/ADHD might need higher doses for effectiveness.

The doctors who have shared this info with us are not sure if this is because of the ADD/ADHD medication or another reason but definitely worth discussing with your doctor if you have ADD/ADHD. There is also some new preliminary research indicating using caution in those with a history of a traumatic brain injury (TBI)If you have had a TBI discuss this with your doctor.

9. You should also have your vitamin B12 checked. Some providers have started giving a Vitamin B12 shot to patients that are late responders and have found it has increased their results for depression infusions.

*** If anything feels off or not right after an infusion please don't hesitate to be in touch with your healthcare provider. Never hesitate to contact them. That is what they are there for. Make sure you have a phone number to reach your provider during hours when the office is closed.***

CHAPTER 3

Choosing a Provider

~~~~~~~

How do I choose the best provider?

1. When picking a place to get your infusions done, confirm that a physician or CRNA* is on site at all times during Infusions.

2. Look for a place that provides a comfortable and relaxed atmosphere, has comfortable recliners or full beds for infusions, and maintains a quiet space for patients.

3. Don't be afraid to ask how much experience they have in giving Ketamine infusions. Approximately how many patients have they infused? What has their success rate been? One of the best things you can ask is how the clinician decided to start doing ketamine infusions. From this question, you can usually tell if he or she has the "heart" for this sort of medicine, or if they are simply there giving you a medication without thought. This may sound strange, but I believe the person involved in your infusions should have a genuine interest in this type of work and understand exactly how

it works, how to titrate the dosage, and how to handle complications.

Ask them questions such as:

1. Do they have emergency equipment on hand in case it is needed? Have they ever had an emergency? How was it handled if yes.

2. Ask how patients are monitored during the infusions; how often are vital signs checked?

3. How long are patients observed for after infusions?

4. Are the infusions ran "on a pump" meaning the rate is closely controlled by a machine?

5. Do they make you have a companion or a sitter in the room during Infusions? (This is more common for pain patients who are receiving longer infusions.)

6. What is their bathroom policy during infusions? Do they allow you to get up with help during the infusion or do they have a bedside commode or bedpan? (This is usually more for pain patients who are getting 4 hour infusions.)

7. How can the doctor be reached after hours in an emergency?

What is a CRNA? Certified Registered Nurse Anesthetist are nurses who have continued on for extensive training in anesthesia. CRNA's are used in hospitals and outpatient surgery centers all over the United States to administer anesthesia to patients undergoing procedures.

CHAPTER 4

Ketamine Dosing and Typical Protocols

~~~~~~~~

A very common question asked, is there a specific dose for Ketamine?

Ketamine is a very unique drug in the way it works. There is no specific dose that works for everyone, whether patients are receiving it for pain or for mental health. Based on your situation, medications, and overall health status, your doctor will work with you to find the dose that works for you.

What dose do most doctors start their depression patients at?

Most of the studies have shown that a minimum dose of 0.5 mg per kg of patient's weight is necessary to see a response to Ketamine for depression. Most doctors will begin at that dose and slowly raise it until the effective dose for you is found. Be aware that there are, however, some clinics that do not titrate dosage beyond the 0.5 mg/kg.

What dose do most docs start their pain patients at?

For outpatient pain infusions, Pain patients should be started at a minimum of 1 milligram per kilogram of your body weight. It should be slowly raised up from there assuming there are no contraindications to do so; doses below that will have little to no effects for pain.

For inpatient pain infusions it works a little differently, since inpatient infusions are continuous over 24 hours a day usually for five days the first doses are quite low and slowly worked up to about a total of 75 to 80mg an hour. Since the total number will end up being very high, it works out equivalently to the same amount of total Ketamine approximately as given during the higher dose outpatient infusions.

How is the Ketamine given?

Ketamine should only be given as an IV infusion for pain patients.

For patients being treated for mental health Ketamine can be given as an IV infusion or as an intramuscular injection. There is also now a different form of Ketamine, a nasal spray, which we will discuss more a little later.

We do not recommend getting Ketamine IV push other than when administered in the operating room by a trained anesthesia provider. (This is when the entire dose of Ketamine is given all at once.) If a person is awake during this it can cause sudden and abrupt disassociation which can be a scary experience.

Ketamine Administration Protocols:

Multiple studies have shown that one single dose of Ketamine by itself will do little to help pain or depression. The first infusions need to be given as a set and then maintained with ongoing boosters. How often you will need boosters is something that will be determined by you and your doctor after your initial infusions begin to wear off. The average is anywhere from two to six months some patients have even gone up to a year between boosters but that is pretty unusual. Will I need boosters for the rest of my life? Remember in the beginning of the book how we said that Ketamine is a treatment and not a cure? Well just like any other treatment in order for the Ketamine to keep working for you you will need to keep on getting infusions. The good news is that many people have found as time went on they have been able to go longer in between infusions and researchers are working on new drugs that may help extend the benefits of Ketamine infusions.

Ketamine works on certain receptors called NMDA receptors in the brain. (They are finding now that there may be other receptors involved as well.) Ketamine causes a temporary reset of these receptors. Initially multiple infusions are needed to help this temporary reset occur. The reset then wears off after a while and you need to go back again for a booster to cause the temporary reset once again.

The following protocols may vary slightly depending on what your provider does but these are the protocols most doctors are using at this time.

Pain Protocol:

For pain patients there are 2 common initial infusion protocols used:

1. Outpatient High Dose Initial Infusions. These will be given over a total of 5 or 10 days depending on your type of pain. They are given 5 days in a row over 4 hours each day then a break is given for the weekend and

infusions are resumed for another 5 days if you are doing a 10 day initial protocol. Clinics typically do between 5-10 infusions.

2. Inpatient 24 hours a day low dose infusions. There are very few places unfortunately that still are offering the inpatient infusions. These infusions are usually given over 5 to 7 days.

Depression Protocol: For depression there are also two different protocols being used:

1. This was the original protocol: Six initial infusions given every other day over two weeks. Booster schedule will then be determined between your doctor and you.

2. The new protocol was developed very recently is given more spread out,

•   2 Infusions week 1,

•   2 Infusions week 2,

•   1 Infusion week 3,

•   1 Infusion week 4.

•   Booster number 1 scheduled 2 weeks after week 4.

• Booster number 2 scheduled 2 weeks after that.

• Booster number 3 one month later. Then continue with monthly boosters and discuss with your doctor slowly trying to increase the time in between boosters until you figure out what schedule keeps you stable.

These are the protocols that have been researched and shared by several hundred Ketamine providers who have done thousands of infusions. These guidelines are not set in stone. Work closely with your providers to come up with a plan that works for you.

Maintenance Ketamine for at home use, some providers will prescribe a form of Ketamine called a 'troche' that you place in your mouth between the teeth and cheek until it melts or a generic Ketamine nasal spray for use in between infusions. These are much more mild forms of Ketamine as oral and nasal Ketamine are not well absorbed by the body. They do help to increase the time needed in between infusions for some people.

Some doctors will not prescribe them because they are afraid of abuse Since they are so poorly absorbed these low dose forms of Ketamine should not cause any type of disassociation or vivid dreaming like the infusions do which should not make people want to use it for abuse. They may cause some dizziness. It is not recommended to drive after taking a troche or nasal spray for several hours afterwards.

Spravato (also called Esketamine) Nasal Spray is a new form of Ketamine spray made by Janssen Pharmaceuticals. It was created by modifying the original ketamine molecule and, thus, creating a "new" substance. Patients do report a mild form of disassociation while using it. It must be administered in a doctor's office and the patients must be taking another antidepressant along with it. It is only used for mental health diagnoses and will not work for pain as the dose is much to low to be effective for pain.

CHAPTER 5

Adverse Reactions

~~~~~~~

Ketamine overall is a very safe drug. However any drug can have side effects or cause adverse reactions in some people.

The following are the most common side effects experienced,

1. Nausea during the infusions which may continue for several hours afterwards.

2. Lightheadedness and/or dizziness (This can last for a few hours afterwards, which is why you should not drive for 24 hours post infusion. If receiving high dose pain infusions this can last for several days afterwards and is completely normal.)

3. Double vision or blurry vision. Again this is only caused by the very high dose infusions and can last for several hours post infusion.

4. Mood swings and mild anxiety can occur post infusion until the Ketamine has a chance to do its work in the brain.

5. Lucid dreaming or disassociation is normal during Infusions and many providers believe it is a sign the Ketamine is working. (we will discuss this more in another chapter.)

6. High blood pressure which returns to normal post-infusion.

Rare or very Rare possible side effects,

1. Worsening of Bipolar Symptoms or Mania. The current recommendation for people with Bipolar is to treat them during a depressive stage to help prevent possible worsening of mania.

2. Elevated liver enzymes is a rare side effect of Ketamine infusions. (It is more likely to occur in patients who take opiates, drink alcohol, or take a lot of Tylenol.) This is one reason it is recommended to have blood work done to check liver enzymes prior to starting Infusions. You can ask your primary care doctor to order them for you. If your liver enzymes are elevated work with your doctor to find out the cause and help bring them back to normal levels. Once they normalize you can get infusions with continued monitoring of your enzyme levels.

3.   Worsening of Interstitial Cystitis (IC) or other bladder problems. We know Ketamine can be harsh on certain cells in the bladder. If you have a history of bladder issues before starting infusions see your urologist for a baseline cystoscopy and discuss ways to protect the bladder with your urologist. (See IC protocol at the end of the book for more information on this.)

4.   Elevated Intraocular Pressure. According to the literature Ketamine in high doses can cause increased intraocular pressure which returns to normal after infusions. If you have a pre-existing condition that causes an increase in intraocular pressure make sure and get clearance from your ophthalmologist prior to having high dose Ketamine Infusions.

5.   Serotonin Syndrome. Most of the literature says that Ketamine does not affect serotonin levels and so should not cause serotonin syndrome. There seems to be one or two possible reports of someone getting serotonin syndrome while also getting Ketamine. It may have been from one of the other drugs they were on however so I only mention it here for awareness.

*** Remember these are side effects that are known. Always be in touch with your doctor or go to the ER if you experience a severe side effect of Ketamine or any medication.***

CHAPTER 6

What to Expect During the Infusion Experience and How to Mentally Prepare for Your Infusion

~~~~~~~~

Everyone experiences their Ketamine infusions a little differently. Ketamine causes what doctors call a "dissociative state".

What does this mean exactly? The word disassociation according to the dictionary means, "disconnection and lack of continuity between thoughts, memories, surroundings, actions, and identity."

To us that is a terrible description of what Ketamine feels like. We would describe it more as causing one to enter a very vivid dream state. During my wife's infusions she is aware of who she is. She sees colors, shapes, characters, and faces. She finds that her music guides her through her infusions. She says she does feel like the bed or chair moves during her infusions. In fact she calls it her magic carpet ride. We think the best way to describe a Ketamine infusion is like being on a 3D ride at an amusement park.

Can an infusion experience be scary? Why do some people say they "freaked out" during their infusions?

The answer is yes you can have a scary infusion experience occasionally but that is why preparation is key to a good infusion experience. By reading this book you have taken the first step in preparing yourself to make your infusions a pleasant experience.

What causes a scary infusion experience? A few things can cause this, the Ketamine being given too rapidly, the dose being too high for you, and not mentally preparing prior to your infusion.

How do I mentally prepare for my infusions?

1. The day before your infusion, limit social media (except for cat videos, those are okay!)

2. Watch only happy things on TV and do not listen to the news.

3. Use meditation, visualization, or happy mantras to prepare your thoughts. Right before the infusion starts say your happy mantra several times so it is in your mind or visualize the places that make you the most happy and keep that in your mind. Look online for some free

websites that have mediations or mantras you can use to help you prepare.

4. You may want to listen to music. Get your music ready. Find the music that makes you personally feel happy. Whether it is music with words or without find the music that uplifts you and connects with you. It doesn't matter if it is music from your childhood or music that you enjoy now listen to what makes you feel the best.

5. Wear an eye mask and headphones during your infusions to limit outside stimuli that could influence your mindset during your infusion. You want to keep calm and relaxed during infusions if you have someone staying in the room with you ask them not to talk on the phone and not to talk to you unless you ask for reassurance. The calmer and more pleasant the environment the better your infusion will be.

6. All of these are simply suggestions. Ketamine will affect your senses and will affect them all differently. Some patients experience more audible effects than visual, and the other way around. There have been patients who can't handle the pressure of headphones, so earbuds were a better choice. You will

never know what works for you until you are in that moment. I know one physician who will tell her patients that "ketamine will let you know what you want."

What happens if I have a scary infusion experience?

If you are in the middle of your infusion and realize it is getting scary or upsetting first try and redirect your thoughts away from what is upsetting you. Sometimes skipping to the next song on your device can help with that. If that doesn't work ask your provider to try and slow the infusion rate slightly and see if that helps. For mental health infusions discuss with your provider before the infusion starts how they handle if a patient is having a bad infusion experience.

Do they add a benzodiazepine such as versed if you get very agitated? (Remember it is better to avoid benzodiazepines but if you really need it ask for it.)

Afterwards when you have recovered discuss with your provider the best ways to optimize your infusion experience Try and analyze what caused it. Did you see something on TV the day before that upset you? Was this your first time at a higher dose and it made your dreams more vivid? Try and figure out with your provider the cause and see what can be done to prevent it next time.

Just because you had one scary experience does not mean each one will be scary. In fact, every infusion will be different than the last. My wife had one very scary experience and it was before we knew the importance of mental prep beforehand. Now since doing her mental prep every time she has not had it again and she has come to really enjoy her infusions.

What should I expect when my infusion is over for the day?

Once your infusion ends, if you have had a lower dose for mental health, you will usually be pretty awake and alert within a few minutes and will be ready to go home and relax. You must not drive after infusions and all clinics require a driver come to pick you up. Many clinics require the driver sign you out into their care.

If you had the higher dose infusions for pain it can take about 15 to 20 minutes to wake up and you will probably be sleepy and want to rest and sleep most of the day afterwards. If you use a cane or have issues with mobility consider getting a wheelchair to use to go home after your infusion as you may be very dizzy afterwards and have trouble keeping your balance with a cane.

Whether you had high or low dose you may experience dizziness and nausea post infusion which is why you should not drive for at least 12 hours post infusion or for the amount of time your provider instructs you. Expect to go home and rest after infusions.

What can I eat or drink to help with my post infusion recovery? Many providers recommend a protein shake post infusion. Hydration with water is very important post infusion. Some people find a packet of a Vitamin C supplement helps them recover. If getting high dose pain infusions eat lightly afterwards as you may experience some nausea until you see how you feel. Nausea is more common after the high dose infusions though occasionally people will complain of some nausea after the low dose ones. Ginger capsules can help with post infusion nausea. If you keep having post infusion nausea some doctors will give you a prescription for an anti nausea medication such as zofran. Some providers recommend dramamine to help. Speak with your provider to see what they recommend.

CHAPTER 7

What to Bring to My Infusions and Instructions for Eating and Drinking Beforehand

~~~~~~~~

Many providers ask their patients not to eat anywhere from 4 to 12 hours before their infusion depending on whether they are high or low dose. Ketamine can cause nausea and vomiting so definitely discuss this with your provider and find out their policy.

For inpatient infusions you will find that you don't have much appetite during your infusions. Bring protein shakes with you to help you keep up your strength.

We also recommend pain patients have protein shakes on hand if they are doing their initial 5 or 10 day treatments as you won't feel very hungry during them and will sleep a lot of the time in between the infusions. In fact, it's not unusual for patients receiving pain infusions on consecutive days to become dehydrated if extra fluids aren't given by the clinic. Sometimes, patients simply don't feel like eating or drinking after such high doses.

What to bring to my infusions?

1. Music player and headphones (If you've found this works for you.)

2. Eye mask

3. Sunglasses to wear after your infusion on the way to the car as your eyes can be light-sensitive.

4. Soft blanket.

5. A neck pillow or a regular pillow (if you want your own as most places will offer one).

6. Wear comfortable clothes and slip off shoes so you can take them off during your infusion.

7. Some patients bring and wear their own robes over their clothes.

Will I be allowed to use the restroom during my infusion?

Most places giving high dose infusions will not let you get up to use the restroom. Some places ask you to wear a Depends. Some places will give you a bedpan or a bedside commode. For low dose infusions ask your provider what their policy is.

Constipation: For those getting infusions multiple days in a row, constipation can be an issue. Between the Ketamine, Zofran, and Magnesium they all can be very constipating. A few doctors are known to give a medication called Movantik which some say helps. We have found daily Miralax, about 1-2 capfuls keeps things on track. Making sure to hydrate more in between infusions is extremely important as well. If you are having severe issues with constipation and have not gone in a few days make sure and let your provider know as you do not want to become impacted. If you haven't gone in a number of days and begin to get severe stomach pain go to the ER if you cannot get things moving by yourself. Always keep in contact with your provider and let them know what is going on.

CHAPTER 8

Tolerance to Ketamine

~~~~~~

I have heard people build tolerance to Ketamine over time and it can stop working for them is this true?

Unfortunately, this is true for some people. There are people who were getting infusions for 15 years and it stopped working for them.

What causes tolerance and how can we prevent ourselves from developing tolerance quickly and have many years of effectiveness from our infusions?

No one knows exactly what causes tolerance to Ketamine over time but there are things to help prevent or delay this.

1. Ask your doctor to work with you to find the lowest effective dose that works for you and then only raise the dose a small amount when it stops working for you.

2. Spread infusions out as far as you can tolerate without losing the effectiveness of them.

3. Avoid taking drugs that decrease the benefits of Ketamine infusions.

4. If using a take-home form of Ketamine, such as troches or nasal spray, use the lowest effective dose and spread it out as much as possible. Try only taking it on an as needed basis a few times a week. (Discuss with your doctor before making any medication changes.)

5. If you find the effects of Ketamine starting to decrease then discuss with your doctor trying a short break from Ketamine for a few months and then starting again.

CHAPTER 9

Combination Therapy for Mental Health

~~~~~~~

Most of the studies on patients treated with Ketamine for mental health have found the best results with combined therapy of an antidepressant and Ketamine infusions.

Often antidepressants that didn't work or only worked a little will work better after Ketamine treatments have been initiated. Very often lower doses of the antidepressant is needed.

Which antidepressant works best with Ketamine? Many providers have reported that the combination of Wellbutrin and Ketamine seem to work well together but that is up to you and your provider to decide what will work best for you.

Lithium has been found to be a very good mood stabilizer to use with Ketamine as Lamictal and Latuda both can block the effects of Ketamine.

Besides medication, therapy, is also key to success with Ketamine infusions. Even if therapy has not been that successful in the past it is important to try it along with infusions. When I've convinced others to give therapy a try after they undergo infusions, 100% of them have said therapy was then more effective and an entirely different experience.

Some people have also had success with EMDR, TMS, and other combination therapies with Ketamine. Many clinics offer ketamine assisted psychotherapy, but finding a therapist trained to do therapy with ketamine is still limited.

Mood Monitor an online site used to keep track of moods along with your infusions. It helps you decide when you should go in for your booster infusions and helps you keep track of your mood daily. If your provider is not using Mood Monitor I highly recommend asking them to look into signing up for it.

Keeping a journal can also be an important part of Ketamine therapy to help you note subtle improvements in mood as Ketamine begins to work. You should write in your journal as soon as you get up in the morning, or whatever part of the day is the most consistent for you. Write down exactly what you are feeling as soon as you wake up and then again right before bedtime. At the end of the week review your entries to see how you were feeling throughout the week.Use this to discuss with your provider any changes in therapies you might need to make. (If you have OCD and find that you begin to obsess over your journaling then this is not a good method for you.)

Join a local support group or find online support through Facebook or other social media. Ketamine groups are a great way to connect and share your experiences and stories.

CHAPTER 10

The Mindset

~~~~~~~

From all of our talking with people over the years since starting this Ketamine journey we have found one repeating theme over and over.

If you go into your infusions believing they won't be successful for you then they won't be!!!

Ketamine's effects can be very subtle in the beginning for many people. Some people are lucky and feel amazing the day after their infusions are done but for the majority of us, Ketamine works more subtly.

Initially we may feel worse. We may experience a post infusion flare up of our pain or depression. Try and stay positive the infusions can take 2 to 3 weeks to kick in. Some providers want patients to give up if they don't feel results after 3 or 4 infusions. Coming from someone's wife, who after every set of infusions it takes a good two weeks for it to kick in, we say don't give up! We have even heard of cases that have taken up to 4 weeks to kick in after the initial setup; that however is rare.

Ketamine is cumulative. You must receive regular treatments for it to continue to work. The changes can be small and subtle at first.

Pain patients as you start to feel better don't go from zero to sixty overnight. Start to move more slowly. Try and do some physical therapy if you can. We know of many patients that feel so much better, they easily over-do it too soon!

For mental health patients, get out of the house. Go for a walk outside if the weather is nice or somewhere indoors if it is not. Get a coffee with a friend. Do something small every day that brings you pleasure. Essentially, do the things that are generally healthy for everyone: sunshine, good nutrition, stress relief, exercise, etc.

Work on making small positive changes daily. Yes there will be bad days but try to focus on the good ones as much as you can.

And remember there is always hope. If Ketamine is not working for you then hopefully tomorrow another new drug will be released that works for you!

Wishing you sweet Ketamine dreams and much success with your infusions!

ADDENDUM:

Bladder Protection Protocol

~~~~~~~

Ketamine is harsh on the cells of the bladder. People with Interstitial Cystitis have reported some issues with bladder pain or frequent urination after repeated infusions. In order to protect the bladder during Ketamine infusions and lessen any bladder side effects I have worked with a urologist to develop a protocol that helps reduce side effects using supplements and one prescription medication. The protocol consists of the following over the counter supplements. Please check with your own personal provider before using any of these supplements.

1. Aloe Vera Gel Capsules 3 times daily

2. Chondroitin Sulfate 600mg nightly at bedtime

3. Hyaluronic Acid 200mg nightly at bedtime

4. Astaxanthin 12mg at bedtime

5. Half hour prior to Infusions, 2 tablets of Prelief (You can also take prelief prior to taking troches or using

nasal spray, or with any food that makes your bladder sensitive.)

6. For patients diagnosed with Interstitial Cystitis ask your provider about a prescription medication called Uribel which you can take half an hour prior to your Infusions in addition to the other supplements to help reduce the chance of bladder issues post infusion.

Discuss with your provider and ask for an extra 500cc of IV fluid at the end of your infusion. Hydrate very well the day before and the day after your infusions.

About the Author

This work is a compilation of the knowledge of myself and my wife since she began her Ketamine journey in 2011. This book has been 5 years in the making. My wife is a disabled nurse practitioner who has been getting Ketamine infusions for her CRPS and Fibromyalgia since the beginning of 2015. She started reading medical journals and learned as much as she could about Ketamine for chronic pain in 2011 when she first heard it was being used for CRPS. We started exploring the possibility of her getting Ketamine infusions and she was accepted into a research study in 2015. After getting infusions people started connecting with her and asking her for advice about their infusions. We have gotten input on Ketamine infusions from many providers around the world. My wife and I have spent many years researching ketamine and talking to hundreds of patients and physicians about this miraculous treatment in an effort to navigate our own journey with ketamine and it's treatment potential. Fortunately, we finally decided our experience was too valuable not to share with the world. Where her voice may be limited due to her chronic illnesses, mine takes over to encourage you to explore the entirely new, fascinating world of ketamine as a treatment option for chronic pain or refractory mental health conditions.